The Stress Hormone Cortisol

In Chronic Excess, It Can Be the Root Cause of Several Medical Conditions

RON KNESS

Copyright © 2016 Ron Kness

All rights reserved.

ISBN-13: 978-1539785989

ISBN-10: 153978598X

Contents

Disclaimer

We hope you enjoy reading our report however we do suggest you read our disclaimer. All the material written in this report is provided for informational purposes only and is general in nature.

Every person is a unique individual and what has worked for some or even many may not work for you. Any information perceived as advice by must be considered in light of your own particular set of circumstances.

The author or person sharing this information does not assume any responsibility for the accuracy or outcome of your use of the content.

Every attempt has been made to provide well researched and up to date content at the time of writing. Now all the legalities have been taken care of, please enjoy the content.

See your healthcare professional before starting any diet or exercise program!

Stress and Cortisol Resistance

Stress and High Blood Pressure

An Italian research suggests that even mild stress is enough to cause an increase in blood pressure which in turn impairs the functioning of the cardiovascular system. How do we prevent this from happening?

Check out the following tips:

- Get enough sleep.
- Develop your time management skills.
- Eat a healthy well-balanced diet.
- Learn to let go of things beyond your control.
- Develop your sense of gratitude.
- Participate in Yoga, Taichi or transcendental meditation.

A person who is under excessive stress is often described as someone who is always working "under the gun". This expression should be a fair indicator that too much exposure to stress is a big threat to a person's health and well-being.

Repeated studies expose the correlation between stress and ill-health, and why chronic stress is such an important health problem. Cortisol is a type of glucocorticoid hormone. Along with adrenaline, it is one of the main hormones responsible for stress responses.

Adrenaline Hormone

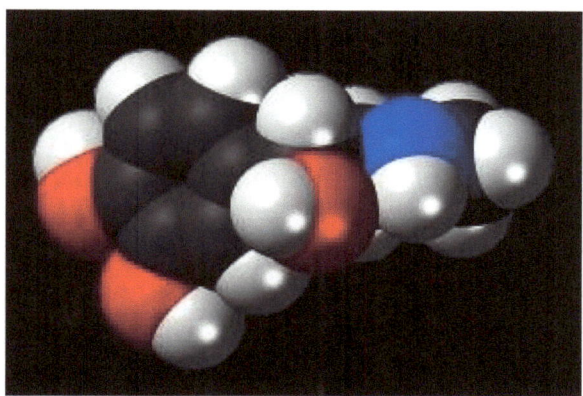

The Role of Cortisol as a Stress Hormone

The actions of cortisol in the human body are quite complex. As a primary stress hormone it not only acts directly on the body, but also acts indirectly by activating other hormones, each with a critical role to perform.

In a healthy person with a healthy cycle consisting of a stress incident followed by an adequate rest and recovery phase, cortisol has a major function of instigating homeostasis, or returning the body to normal after being exposed to stress. This is enacted largely through the triggering of secondary hormones.

The recovery phase following an acute stress incident is critical for the prevention of developing chronic stress. Chronic stress develops when persistent stress causes stress hormones, including cortisol, to remain constantly elevated in the body. In this all too common situation, cortisol remains awash in the body at high levels for long periods of time. Unfortunately in today's world, this is happening a lot.

Chronic Stress and Cortisol Resistance

As is usual in any organism subjected to an excess of almost anything, the receptors become dulled or resistant to the action of that product. In this case the cells and glands that should respond to cortisol will have a greatly reduced response, which in turn means reduced activation of vital secondary hormones.

It has been well-noted that persons suffering from chronic stress have correspondently high levels of cortisol in their system. This correlation led many to make the connection that the excess cortisol was the direct culprit for many of the symptoms of chronic stress.

This is confusing and contradictory, knowing that a primary role of cortisol is to return the body to a normal state following a stressful incident. Recent studies have concluded that the problem with persistent excess cortisol is actually one of resistance.

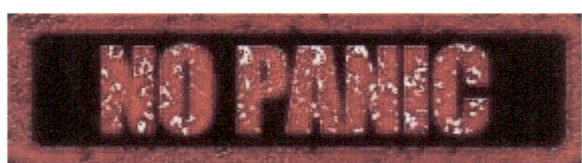

This means that problems occur not so much as a reaction to cortisol, but as a non-reaction to it, caused by resistance. Of course this is still a result of too much cortisol in the system for extended periods, which in turn results from unabated chronic stress.

Stress, Glucocorticoid Resistance and the Common Cold

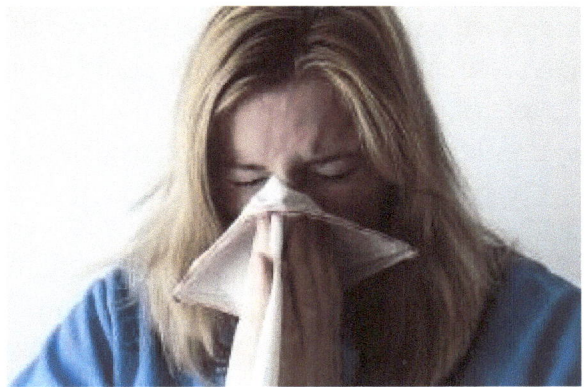

A particular research study published in the Proceedings of the National Academy of Sciences had two objectives.

The first one was to determine whether stress can cause cortisol resistance while the second objective was to determine whether cortisol resistance increases a person's risk of acquiring an infection such as a common cold.

The study had 276 healthy volunteers whose levels of stress, BMI, race, age, sex and glucocorticoid resistance or GCR were thoroughly assessed at the start of the research.

The volunteers were exposed to rhinovirus (i.e. the kind of virus that causes common colds), quarantined and observed for five days.

At the end of the study, researchers found that those volunteers who had recent exposure to an event that contributes to long-term stress developed glucocorticoid resistance which also put them at higher risk of developing a common cold.

Cortisol Resistance and Increased Levels of Inflammation

Another study was conducted which was aimed at determining whether cortisol resistance could cause increased levels of inflammation. This time 79 volunteers had virus exposure and were monitored for five days.

The results showed that those volunteers who were found to have glucocorticoid resistance had more proinflammatory cytokines, which promote systemic inflammation. This study challenged a current perception that stress directly causes disease through elevated cortisol levels.

This most recent scientific literature proposed that the "sensitivity of the cells to cortisol" is more important than the "absolute levels" of cortisol in determining how stress-induced cortisol levels leads to diseases.

When Stress Causes Runaway Inflammatory Response

One of the very important functions of cortisol is to turn off the inflammatory response. For example, when you catch a cold or your skin is wounded, you will immediately suffer from an inflammation which serves as your body's natural protective response to an injury or illness.

Acute inflammation is beneficial in the extreme short term as is seals the body against further attack. Soon after you get an injury or disease your body will secrete cortisol and activate its glucocorticoid receptors to be able to turn off the inflammatory response.

However, this procedure does not occur as efficiently as it should in stressed individuals. Researchers discovered that chronically stressed individuals produced cortisol when responding to a disease or injury but subsequently failed to activate their glucocorticoid receptors. As a result, stressed individuals can have a "runaway" inflammatory response.

Stress causes high levels of cortisol but chronic stress helps subsequently develop cortisol resistance that causes increased susceptibility to disease. Cortisol resistance is common to those who have depression and to the majority of those who are chronically stressed. Cortisol resistance is a much bigger contributor to the development of disease than previously recognized.

To reiterate, it is not the high levels of cortisol that contributes to the development of a particular disease but rather it is the "insensitivity" of the cellular receptors to cortisol that increases an individual's vulnerability to disease. These findings reinforce the science behind the confirmed link between stress and susceptibility to disease.

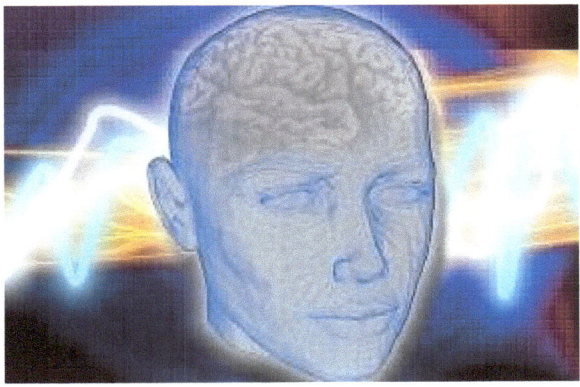

The bottom line for anyone suffering the effects still remain the same. It is necessary for improved health to reduce the persistent levels of cortisol in the system.

Subjects can take a two-pronged approach to reducing cortisol levels:

- Firstly – by reducing the stress that is the root cause of the problem, either by eliminating the stressors, or by improving the ability to cope with them. A reduced emotional response to any stressor will mean a reduced chemical reaction and less cortisol release.
- Secondly – there are known behavioral and dietary 'hacks' that assist the mind and body to reduce the release of cortisol into the system. There are also some common behavioral and dietary habits that greatly increase cortisol production.

A combination of both approaches will provide the fastest path to overcoming the distressing symptoms of chronic stress.

Habits That Elevate Cortisol Levels

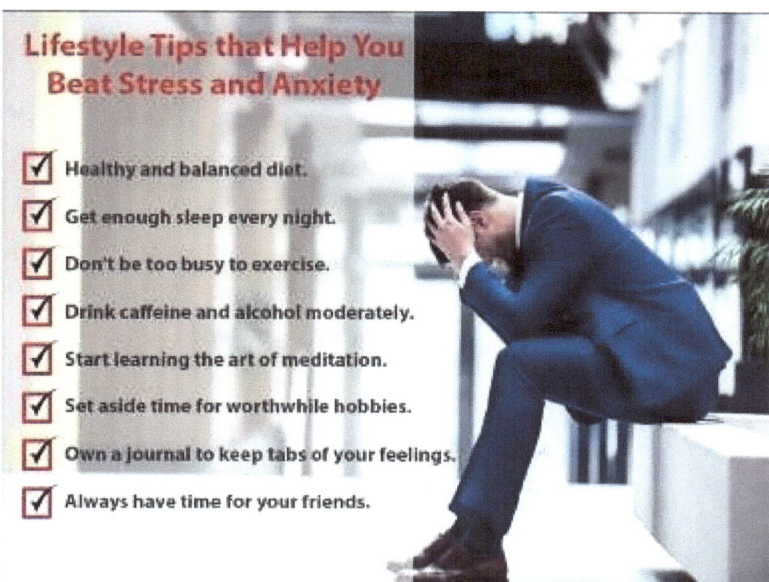

Lifestyle Tips that Help You Beat Stress and Anxiety

- ☑ Healthy and balanced diet.
- ☑ Get enough sleep every night.
- ☑ Don't be too busy to exercise.
- ☑ Drink caffeine and alcohol moderately.
- ☑ Start learning the art of meditation.
- ☑ Set aside time for worthwhile hobbies.
- ☑ Own a journal to keep tabs of your feelings.
- ☑ Always have time for your friends.

Cortisol is at its highest level in the morning. Once cortisol is secreted, it affects a great many of the body's processes and functions. It not only affects several metabolic processes but it can also affect a person's immune response and memory.

After a stressful event many people engage in varying forms of substance abuse for emotional relief. For example, they may want to indulge in an excess of alcohol or even drugs.

Bingeing on these and caffeinated beverages does not help at all. It is a common belief that one of the best ways to overcome stress is to release it with large amounts of caffeine, alcohol or both. This is incorrect.

Ironically, consuming these substances will actually stimulate the body to produce even more cortisol.

Alcohol intake was found to elevate cortisol levels much more than any stress stimuli. The continued elevation of cortisol levels caused by alcohol, caffeine and also a lack of sleep, can further compound the effects of stress that sufferers are trying to defeat.

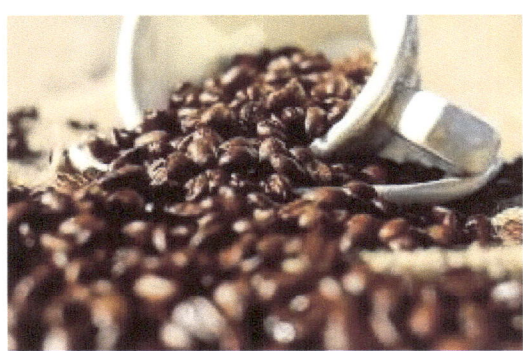

Caffeine and Increased Cortisol Levels

Drinking several cups of coffee or any caffeinated beverage in a single day can cause an increase in cortisol production. These elevated levels occur irrespective of the type of stressor involved or the individual's gender.

Although the extent of the connection between caffeine and cortisol has not yet been fully studied, these findings indicate a positive relationship between increased caffeine intake and high cortisol levels which can also be exacerbated with the introduction of different forms of stressors.

When a lack of sleep is compounded with increased caffeine intake, the negative effects of stress are reinforced as more stress hormones are released in an effort to support an already stressed and struggling system.

Sleep Deprivation, Alcohol Intake and Stress

A study taken on stressed students revealed that their sleep deprivation combined with their increased caffeine or alcohol intake produced high cortisol levels. The high consumption of alcohol and caffeine was triggering an increase in cortisol production, thereby further aggravating their stress responses.

The researchers found that sleep deprivation raised the students' plasma cortisol levels by up to 45 percent. Such an increase is enough to cause cognitive impairment, metabolic disruption and compromised immune response.

Tips for Lowering Cortisol Levels

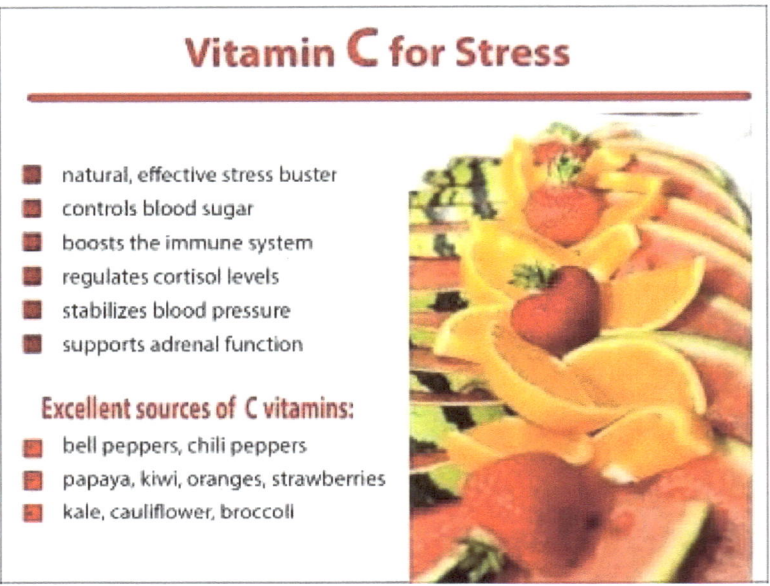

Vitamin C for Stress

- natural, effective stress buster
- controls blood sugar
- boosts the immune system
- regulates cortisol levels
- stabilizes blood pressure
- supports adrenal function

Excellent sources of C vitamins:
- bell peppers, chili peppers
- papaya, kiwi, oranges, strawberries
- kale, cauliflower, broccoli

The production of cortisol in your body is beneficial for regulating your blood pressure and for enhancing your immune response especially during highly stressful moments. Cortisol taps your energy reserves while increasing your body's ability to fight off different kinds of infections.

However, problems begin when a person is chronically stressed. Relentless stress keeps a person's cortisol levels churning in high gear, subverting the supposedly good intentions of the critical hormone.

As a result, the person experiences difficulty sleeping which may further lead to depressed immune response, abnormalities in blood sugar levels and increasing waist lines.

When a person's cortisol levels spike, they will have the tendency to crave calorie-rich foods. This response serves as the body's innate survival tactic for supplying rapid energy such as might be needed to flee from a predator. Of course, such a response is less than helpful if a person is actually stressed over how to beat deadlines in the workplace.

The good news is that solutions to these unneeded heightened cortisol levels are available. Here are some ways to exploit the body's relaxation response and lower your cortisol levels:

Mindfulness Meditation

A study was conducted on 57 individuals who were asked to undergo a meditation retreat. At the same time, they were also taught some stress management skills such as mindful breathing and cultivating one's own positive mental state. At the beginning and end of the study the participants' cortisol levels were also measured through a saliva test.

After their meditation retreat, researchers found out that their mindfulness scores were higher compared to their scores at the start of the study. A significant finding of the study was that as the participants' mindfulness scores increased, their cortisol levels decreased.

Sleep

Lowering your cortisol levels can be as simple as getting enough sleep. If you are among those people who have sleeping problems, look at ways to increase your melatonin.

Melatonin allows you to sleep deeper and longer. It is often recommended for air travelers to help them overcome jet lag and to reset their body clock after moving into different time zones.

Melatonin supplementation is available but it also occurs naturally in foods such as pineapples, oranges and bananas.

Tea

Drinking a cup of tea provides you with L-theanine which is an amino acid that contributes to feelings of relaxation and better sleep.

While all teas may contain some L-theanine research shows that some kinds such as Japanese green tea and gyokuro of tea have higher concentrations of this substance.

Vitamin C

Vitamin C has been one of the most sought after and widely-known nutritional supplements for many years. Its absolute necessity for preventing conditions such as scurvy and its proven efficacy in overcoming infection, colds and flu are well documented. It even became controversial when some experts revealed study results claiming that vitamin C in sufficient dosage can prevent heart diseases and cancer. However, the benefits of vitamin C don't end there.

Researchers have added another reason why people should consider taking vitamin C supplements. This vitamin is being touted as a very effective supplement for alleviating the symptoms of stress and perhaps should be included as part of your stress management plan.

Vitamin C is an Effective Stress Buster

Studies show that those people who had been regularly taking vitamin C supplements and have been eating vitamin C rich foods were found to exhibit far less of the physical and mental signs of stress than those who had low levels of Vitamin C.

One study conducted by German researchers showed that those individuals who were regularly given 1,000 mg of vitamin C had lower levels of measured stress hormones even after being subjected to highly-stressful events such as public-speaking and mathematical calculations.

However, those people who were not given Vitamin C supplementation, experienced increased blood pressure after undergoing the same events.

From these findings, it has been suggested that taking vitamin C supplements are beneficial against the debilitating effects of stress.

Vitamin C Improves the Immune System

Another study showed that vitamin C can help prevent the overproduction of stress hormones in the body. Excessive production of stress hormones in the body contributes to suppression of the immune system. Therefore, a regular intake of vitamin C can lead to improved immune system functionality, as well as reduced susceptibility to many illnesses which are brought about or made worse by too much stress.

This theory was proven when researchers studied marathon runners. Those who regularly took vitamin C were found to be less vulnerable to the common cold and other respiratory illnesses compared to those marathon athletes who ignored this supplement.

Sources of Vitamin C

Vitamin C is very sensitive to air, temperature and water. Steaming, boiling or blanching a vegetable may result in the loss of vitamin C by as much as 25%. Loss may also occur when a vitamin C-rich food undergoes thawing and freezing.

When a vegetable or fruit is cooked for 10-20 minutes, only half of its vitamin C content remains.

Eating fruits and vegetables while they are still raw and fresh is the best way to maximize your vitamin C intake. The following are some of the fruits and vegetables that contain high levels of the vitamin:

- Bell peppers, hot and green chili peppers
- Mustard greens, kale, cauliflower, broccoli
- Papaya, kiwi, orange, strawberries, tangerines.

Vitamin C is best obtained through eating fresh fruits and vegetables. However, taking it as a supplement may also be helpful especially to people who are living in places where fresh fruits and vegetables are scarce or seasonal.

There is no one single magic bullet to prevent or relieve stress. Sufferers need to review all aspects of their life including diet. Using vitamin C in conjunction with other natural stress reduction techniques will help build resilience in mind and body to better cope with your stress.

Swedish Massage

One study showed that indulging in a Swedish massage helps lower an individual's cortisol levels. The study involved 53 participants; 24 of them were asked to indulge in a light-touch massage while the other 29 had Swedish massage for 45 minutes once or twice a week.

After five weeks, those participants who underwent Swedish massage had lower levels of cortisol compared to those who only had light massage.

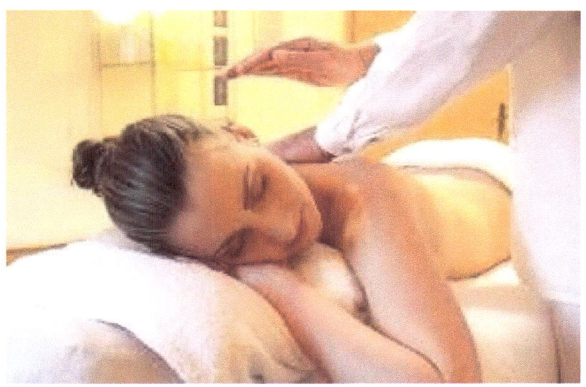

Diet

If you are the kind of person who feels constantly stressed, make sure that what you are eating helps you reduce, not increase, your cortisol levels.

Your daily diet should include good sources of protein such as meat, eggs, poultry, fish and dairy products. You also need your daily dose of omega-3 fatty acids which can be obtained from flax seeds, walnuts, salmon and sardines.

Include more fruits and vegetables in your diet, especially those that contain high amounts of vitamin C as noted earlier which reduces cortisol secretion in the body.

Hypnosis

Hypnosis or hypnotherapy for stress, can serve as a powerful tool to change the way people use their minds. Hypnosis has been found extremely helpful for alleviating stress and anxiety.

Hypnosis refers to the artful manipulation of a person's attention, context and language to be able to establish a temporary belief which can influence a person's behavior and perception. This practice is rooted in a belief that an individual's mind can be manipulated by suggestion, the kind that is powerful enough to affect one's body.

The practice of hypnosis still stirs up debate among some professionals from the more mainstream fields of health and medicine. But, there have been studies conducted to prove its potency in helping people ease their pain and cope with the debilitating effects of stress.

Brain Scan Reveals How Hypnosis Works

Hypnosis has been proven by research conducted in Stanford University which employs the latest and state-of-the-art imaging tools to be able to capture what goes on inside the brain during and after hypnosis. A specialized MRI brain scan revealed decreased activity in two areas of the brain under hypnosis – the one responsible for visual processing and the other one involved in handling conflicts.

Experts say the decreased activity in these two areas explains why a hypnotized brain becomes more accepting to suggestions. It's been shown that hypnotic suggestions are powerful ways to influence brain activity which in turn can also influence an individual's behavior.

How Hypnosis Helps to Combat Stress

Stress and anxiety are emotional health problems and hypnosis dives into the sub-conscious mind. Hypnosis actually gets to the root of the problem, which is a great place to start!

Through the power of suggestion, the mind can tell the body how it should respond to stress. If the mind can tell the body to relax and stay calm during a stressful episode, the body will immediately obey.

Hypnosis is also used to find out what the trigger's for the stress or anxiety problem is. Once the mind is in a deep, relaxed state and all negative thoughts have dissipated, the brain no longer has room for stress to be in it.

Some people like to try self-hypnosis, while others use the help of a trained hypnotherapist. People that have become adept at using self-hypnosis find it easier to reduce their level of anxiety when stressful situations are imminent. It is also through hypnosis that they have learned how to spot situations that trigger a stressful response.

Low Impact Exercise

Exercising is a great way to improve health, feel better and alleviate stress. For some, the very thought of exercising can feel overwhelming and the prospect of engaging in aerobic activity can add to current stress.

The fact is if you engage in exercise, you will feel much more relaxed at the end of it. Working up a sweat can be therapeutic on many levels. Envisioning the source of your stress and then doing something physical to that source, for example shadow-boxing, can be an excellent release.

Getting your heart rate up for an extended period enables your brain to release your 'feel good' endorphins.

Low Impact Exercise Options

Yoga and Pilates are excellent stress relief forms of exercise; particularly if you suffer from joint and muscle pain. Many people have difficulty with high impact exercise. Most people who go to a yoga class for the first time are shocked at how sore they feel the next day. There seems to be this idea that yoga simply consists of light stretching.

These ancient poses engage numerous muscle groups. Taking slow, deep breaths while holding the yoga poses, helps to facilitate a cleansing process within our body, enabling accumulated toxins to release.

Pilates is excellent for toning and sculpting the muscles. These workouts are considered to be moderate intensity. Not only will you become fitter over time, you will possibly shed some weight too. The pace is fairly slow but the importance is doing the exercises correctly and breathing properly in the process. As you notice your body responding in a positive manner, you will be more inclined to keep these workouts up.

Daily Walks

Making time to get outside everyday can make a huge difference in your ability to cope with stress. Reconnecting with fresh air, sunshine and vitamin D, and the vegetation surrounding you is important. Unfortunately, many of us spend no time outdoors anymore. This is a sad human condition.

The majority of our ancestors spent their lives farming or growing a garden, tending to livestock and chopping wood. The need to be outside in nature is something that is in our veins.

Taking time to smell the flowers and chat with your neighbors are positive ways to alleviate stress.

Walking and any exercise helps to get your circulation flowing. Exercise often clears your mind and leaves you feeling invigorated. Not only will your mood be improved, you will most likely have more patience with your spouse and kids.

When you feel good about yourself and your choices, you will naturally be less stressed. When you feel like you are being proactive in living a healthy lifestyle, you will be proud of yourself and how you have incorporated new positive methods for handling stress.

Eating for Improved Cortisol Levels

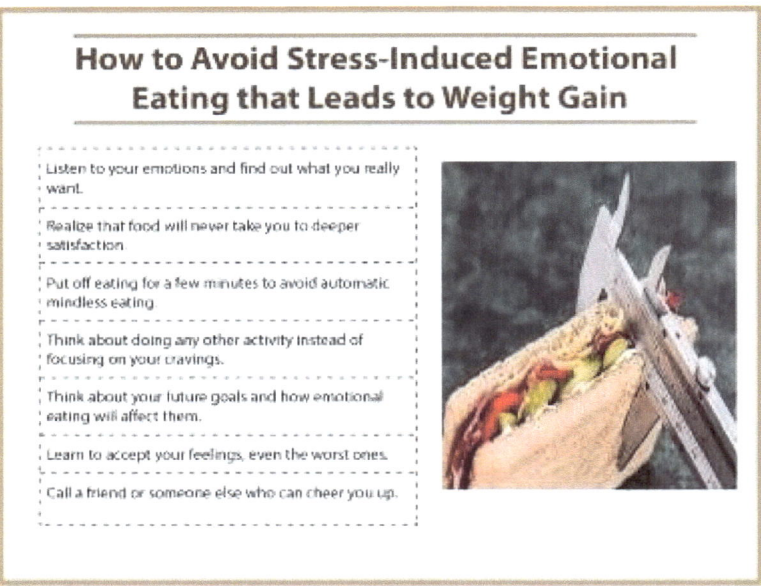

How to Avoid Stress-Induced Emotional Eating that Leads to Weight Gain

Listen to your emotions and find out what you really want.

Realize that food will never take you to deeper satisfaction

Put off eating for a few minutes to avoid automatic mindless eating

Think about doing any other activity instead of focusing on your cravings.

Think about your future goals and how emotional eating will affect them.

Learn to accept your feelings, even the worst ones.

Call a friend or someone else who can cheer you up.

When produced by the adrenal glands in normal levels cortisol provides more strength and is in some ways more powerful than adrenaline.

Cortisol is called the "wake-up-and-tackle-life's-challenges" hormone because it is at its peak in the morning and will slowly subside throughout the day and the evening. If a person has high levels of cortisol they have increased alertness and awareness.

When faced with a highly-stressful situation, cortisol will normally rise above the normal resting level. Problems arise when an individual is chronically exposed to too much stress as their adrenal glands are triggered to produce high levels of cortisol almost without respite.

As a result, they will feel wired all the time and relaxation and recovery may start to become very elusive.

The ideal remedy is to reduce exposure to the events or people causing the stress. For most people this may not be a realistic option, and it is therefore imperative to learn how to better deal with the stressors and implement behaviors to reduce production of excess cortisol.

As part of this program, you can help keep cortisol levels lower by eating the right kind of foods. Check out the following guide to your daily diet for keeping your cortisol within normal levels.

Citrus Fruits

Instead of reaching for sugary treats during stressful times, instead choose oranges, kiwis or any citrus fruits. Vitamin C can help slow down your body's production of cortisol while also quickly clearing it from your bloodstream.

Vitamin C is also beneficial for the prevention of blood pressure spikes that usually occur as part of your body's response to stress.

Omega-3 Fatty Acids

Omega 3 is not only helpful for inhibiting inflammation but it is also great for cortisol reduction. Include omega-3 rich foods in your daily diet such as haddock, flaxseed, mackerel, walnuts, tofu, shrimp and cauliflower.

Microgreens

Microgreens are salad greens picked very young, usually soon after the first leaves have formed. The great thing about microgreens is that they contain higher concentrations of stress-busting vitamin C. Young cilantro and baby red cabbages contain up to six times more vitamin C than their mature versions.

If you have the time and space growing your own microgreens is a good way of bringing nature into your home and of making nutrition just a hand-pick away. If not, they are usually readily available in the produce section of the supermarket, as they are highly sought for their nutritive, taste and garnishing qualities.

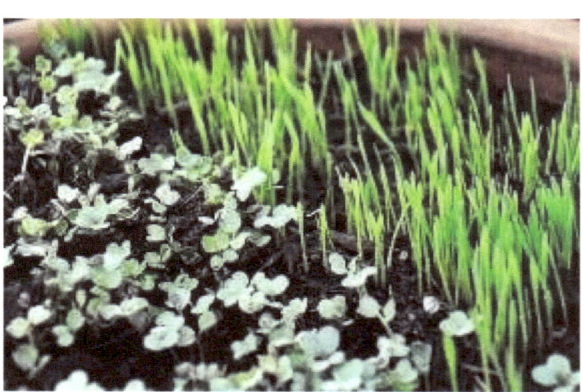

Holy Basil

Holy Basil is known for its ability to function as an adaptogen which is beneficial for enhancing the body's response against mental and physical stress.

Although holy basil cannot alter one's mood, it ensures optimal functioning of the body during stressful times. Several scientific studies have demonstrated the ability of holy basil to reduce the levels of stress hormones specifically cortisol.

Dark Chocolate

If stress causes you to crave for something sweet opt for dark chocolate that contain 70 per cent cocoa. This chocolate helps boost the production of endorphins and serotonin in the brain. Consuming 1.4 ounce of dark chocolates every day for two weeks has been proven effective for lowering one's cortisol levels.

Take care here, as more is not necessarily better!

Protein

Protein from high quality animal meats can greatly reduce cortisol production. Eating 15-30 grams of protein-rich foods every three hours can drastically blunt the production of cortisol in the body. Good sources of protein include turkey and chicken, salmon and tuna, and grass-fed beef and lamb.

Lysine

A study published in the Proceedings of the National Academy of Sciences showed that consumption of lysine-rich foods can help reduce the amount of cortisol in the blood. Dietary sources of lysine include eggs, pork, fish, red meat and poultry.

Conclusion

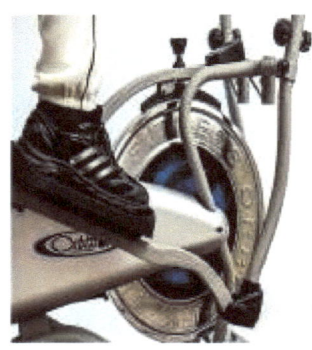

Exercise is a Stress Reliever

Here are more reasons for you to exercise:

- A brain scan of sedentary seniors aged 60-79 showed significant increase in their brain's volume after indulging in aerobic fitness training for six months. This translates to fewer age-related changes that may affect one's ability to cope with stress.

- It boosts your body's production of dopamine and serotonin which promotes improved mood.

- It boosts self-esteem, promotes good sleep, improves energy and lowers risk of dementia, heart disease, type 2 diabetes and stroke.

Cortisol has been given some bad press, mostly due to misunderstandings about its method of operation. In a human who experiences stress cycles as our ancestors did, cortisol is a hormone that performs a magnificent role in dealing with stress and recovering from it.

Unfortunately, the constancy of stress in modern life means that our bodies are subject to more cortisol than nature intended and our cortisol receptors become overwhelmed and resistant to its effects. This means our bodies and our minds are much less capable of dealing with the stress that causes this to happen.

Using the methods discussed here will help to reduce the flood of cortisol released into the body, as part of a program to overcome the crushing symptoms of chronic stress.

Other Relevant Health Books by This Author

If you would like to read more about Senior Health and Fitness, here is a partial list of the titles, CreateSpace links and descriptions from this author:

https://www.createspace.com/6675102

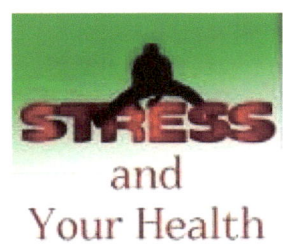

Stress and Your Health

While the word "stress" has many different meanings, as discussed in this publication it refers to the health condition which is all but endemic in modern society. The human body, mind and all its sub-systems developed to deal with the challenges of much more primitive circumstances than we live in now.

Our rapid-response "fight or flight" response system enabled our species to outperform and out-think our way past all others. Collectively our incredible brains have allowed us to live today in a manner that does not require us to engage in the type of activities that made our stress hormones a major asset.

Unfortunately, our physiology has not kept pace with our intellectual development and there is no magic switch to turn off or at least turn down our survival responses.

Today, in civilized societies, we encounter a different manner of struggles and challenges. Even though these situations may not actually be life or death in nature, because of the emotion we attach to our various actions, our minds perceive them as such, and react accordingly.

For many or most people, their bodies and mind are in a constant state of heightened anxiety due to the continually elevated levels of stress hormones in their system. This is chronic stress and its symptoms are broad, varied and can ultimately even be fatal.

We are taught so many things that enable us to live in a social environment with our fellow humans, but too many of us lack knowledge of how to deal with the pressure and stress this can apply. Inability to deal with the causes of stress leads to increased stress and inability to deal with the symptoms of stress can make life seem not worth living.

This publication details some of the signs and symptoms of chronic stress and their damaging effects on our minds and bodies. If you feel stress is negatively impacting your life, make changes. Reduce the causes, or learn to cope with them more appropriately to lessen the impact on you.

https://www.createspace.com/6357470

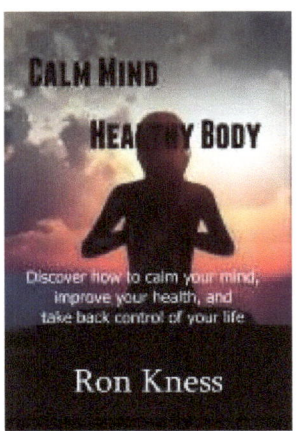

Calm Mind – Healthy Body

Do you ever get the feeling like you're constantly putting out fires? Like life is one massive struggle to stay afloat?

Do you come home from work feeling tired and stressed and without the energy to do anything other than collapse in front of the TV?

Do you always feel like you're just not quite as happy as you think you could/should be?

That's life my friend in today's world. Or at least it's life as many of us have come to know it. In fact though, there's no reason this should necessarily be the case.

The problem is we're always chasing after the gold at the end of the rainbow and in doing so, we end up chasing out tail and take the time to stop and smell the roses.
We're never happy because we're always striving for "the next big thing" and what is coming next.

We're always stressed about what's coming up and we never appreciate what we have here and now until we lose it.

We think the only way to change this is to change our lives. To work harder and longer, which in the end only adds to the problem.

But it's not. The way we change this is from the inside out. We need to change the way we think about our situation and we need to change the way we approach life's problems and the way we enjoy the moment.

And that means taking control of our individual minds.

Once you can do that, you can take back control and you can feel confident, relaxed and happy in the exact same circumstances. Once you can do that, you can start creating the space to actually plot a course and to start changing life for the better. You can stop treading water and actually start swimming.

All very abstract, yes. So far it sounds like a platitude from a bumper sticker.

But stick with me, because this is where the science comes in. And it might just change the way you think about your life, your brain and the interplay between the two.

In this book, we discuss various techniques in which you can use to calm your mind and improve your health.

https://www.createspace.com/6296681

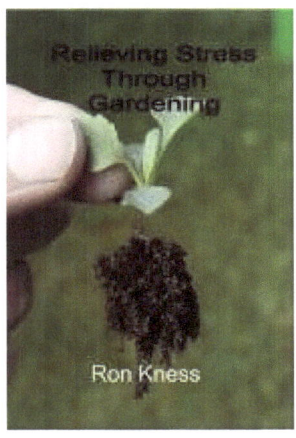

Relieving Stress Through Gardening

Warning: Stress Is Spiraling Dangerously Out of Control and So Is Prescription Drug Abuse

Learn How to Handle Your Stress Through a Natural Solution That Provides Both Mental and Physical Health Benefits!

In "Relieving Stress Through Gardening", you're going to discover an all natural solution that zaps stress and eliminates the need for you to pop pills on a regular basis.

Gardening sounds like a simple activity, but the benefits are both mental and physical in nature. There are vitamins absorbed through the skin from the sun and beneficial bacteria that thrive in the dirt – both of which help diminish your cortisol levels and help you handle whatever comes your way.

In Gardening for Stress Relief, you'll begin to understand…

==> The Scientific Explanation for How Gardening Impacts Your Sleep Cycles and Helps Eliminate Stress Permanently!

==> Why Gardening Trumps Exercise in Helping You Stick to a Program of All Natural Stress Relieving Physical Activity That Sends Cortisol Packing Through Feel Good Hormones!

==> How Gardening Contributes to a Peaceful State of Mind That Carries Over to Your Bedtime Ritual and Removes Stress from Your Sleep Equation!

==> The Precise Way Gardening Puts Your Sleep Cycles Back on Track after They've Been Derailed by Excessive Amounts of Stress!

==> How Gardening Helps Kids Leave the Pressures of the World Behind and Get a Good Night's Sleep!

==> Specific Plants You Can Grow in Your Garden to Help You Relax and Unwind at the End of a Hard Day So You Can Drift Off with Ease!

==> Why Gardening Has Been Called the #1 Sleep Aid that Trumps Prescription Drugs and Contributes to Your Health from Head to Toe!

Once you start gardening, whether it's on a small micro scale or a large plot of land, you'll begin to see immediate changes in the way that you rest each night. You'll be amazed at how the combination of vitamin D, fresh air, peace of mind and low impact physical activity makes you nod off without hesitation.

https://www.createspace.com/6236630

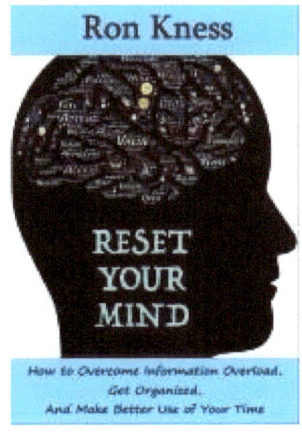

Reset Your Mind

Have you ever thought that maybe you had too much on your plate?

That you'd work better if you had less on your mind?

Imagine how free you'd feel. Much less stressed and able to think clearly for the first time!

Believe it or not, feeling the way you are now is not normal you don't have to be overloaded.

Can You Imagine Working Twice As Fast?

You can by applying what is in our detailed and informative guide that will give you guidance on how YOU can rid yourself of information overload and work more efficiently and effectively.

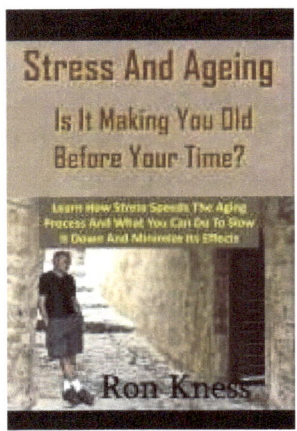

Stress and Ageing

The stress response occurs when external or internal factors cause the body's adrenal glands to put out excess epinephrine, norepinephrine, and cortisol.

These response hormones can result in an increased heart rate, respiratory rate, blood pressure, and blood glucose levels.

A stressor can be anything from having a bad day at the office, relationship issues, physical or emotional distress, financial problems, and a whole host of other things that infiltrate our daily lives, resulting in a stress response.

While stress is normal, too much of it, or too often, can lead to negative effects on your health. In this book we discuss how to recognize stress and how to minimize its effects to keep you from getting old before your time.

About the Author

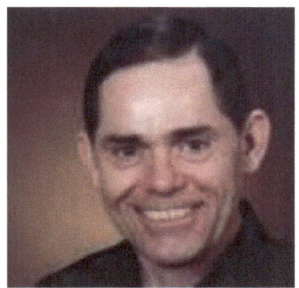

I grew up in Central Minnesota, where my parents owned and operated a fishing resort. Once out of high school I tried a couple of semesters of college, only to quit halfway through the Spring term; I decided at that time that college wasn't for me.

Then I decided to follow my father's previous occupation as an auto mechanic. I graduated from a two-year of vocational training course and worked as a mechanic for five years. While in vocational training, I decided to join the National Guard where I eventually ended up working full-time for 32 years.

So how does all of this relate to writing? In one of my leadership schools, the instructor, who was an English teacher at a juvenile detention center, presented writing to me in a whole new way - a way that started to develop my interest in working with words.

I eventually went back to college on the GI Bill while I was working and earned my Bachelor's degree in Business Administration. Taking a class or two per semester at night and on weekends took me seven years to complete my degree.

Fast forward about 40 years and I now have published over 75 books on Amazon for Kindle, CreateSpace and other publishing platforms.

Besides my own writing, I also ghostwrite ebooks, reports, articles, blogs and do Kindle conversions for clients on a variety of topics.

Today my wife and I are retired from our careers and live in Gold Canyon, AZ. I now write as a retirement business where you'll find me happily sitting in my office typing away on my laptop as I work on my next book or ghostwriting project . . . that is if we are not traveling on a cruise ship - our new-found mode of travel.